vagabond fitness

vagabond fitness

A FIELD MANUAL FOR TRAVELERS

HANK SCHACHTE

ORCA BOOK PUBLISHERS

Canadian Cataloguing in Publication Data
       Schachte, Hank, 1939-
       Vagabond fitness

     ISBN 1-55143-078-9

1. Travelers–Health and hygiene. 2. Exercise.
3. Physical education and training. 1. Title.
GV481.S32 1996   613.7'1'08891   C95-911168-9

Printed and bound in Canada

Orca Book Publishers   Orca Book Publishers
PO Box 5626, Station B   PO Box 468
Victoria, BC Canada   Custer, WA USA
V8R 6S4   98240-0468

PREFACE

It's been a lot of years since I decided to become a writer. Even then I was aware of the experience of my father, who had insisted in his youth that he would never spend his life behind a desk — and then proceeded to do just that.

I grew up in the fifties, when nobody thought too much about the dazzling ease our society had succeeded in providing. I think my father, who was an athlete when young, was a typical casualty of the general inexperience of a motorized public. He suffered a myriad of complaints, though he never smoked nor drank to excess, and loved to work around the yard on weekends. Hospitalized many times for a back ailment, there was almost always a certain amount of physical pain accompanying him, which he endured with cheerful resignation and heating pads, ever eager to plant another shrub or take the scouts hiking. But, when my own back was injured at age nineteen, I wondered if there wasn't something I could do to make a difference.

Over the next fifteen years I tried hundreds of ideas, many borrowed, some deduced: different exercises, routines, yoga and diet. Also, early on I made a deal with myself that for every hour I spent writing I would try to spend an hour outside doing something physical.

At some point during that initial fifteen years of experimentation, in spite of some continuing back problems, I finally seemed to have gotten it right. I developed a routine that worked. After that there were many excursions into less of this and more of that. I found I had to give up some things that felt great but turned out to be contributing to some small problem or other, and I added new things. Also, being something of a minimalist, I have tried to eliminate the unnecessary, until what we have left, it is fair to say, is a distillation.

So I have had a long history of thinking and reading and talking about these things and trying them all out, considering my own body as worthy a guinea pig as any, and the only one with which I could ethically condone experimenting. For encouragement I admit the drawings are faithfully of me and as I write this I am fifty-six and too busy to do much else than this program, which I do whether traveling or not.

What I offer in *Vagabond Fitness* is my accumulated amateur wisdom, approved by experts in the field, a program for the self-reliant. I offer it to you as a gift to a friend.

INTRODUCTION

Modern culture equates value with money, and rarely in this day are major commitments made without the expenditure of rather large sums of money. We also equate time with money. Here again one might expect to invest large sums.

So in its own quiet way, this little book may seem subversive, announcing as it does that we can look after ourselves and achieve healthy fitness with only a modicum of time and essentially no money. But that is, in fact, what it says.

You may have woefully neglected your body, or you may be in good shape. You may be working out already, or be involved with sport. But typically there will be many times in any busy life when you are away from home and your usual routine. You need something more portable, something always with you, a core program, a mental map of your body's actual needs, so you need never feel lost.

Also, no matter who you are, of whatever age and condition, certain processes of time are up and running within you and little by little you will feel their effects. Minimizing these and keeping you happy and pain-free with the least fuss is the thrust of this program.

I take for starters that, like me, you are busy and travel light, maybe light enough not to include sweats or even running shoes, and certainly light enough not to want to be dragging around any of the whole litany of fitness paraphernalia that is out there begging to be purchased. Let *Vagabond Fitness* be your only dedicated extra.

I also assume you are of average health and have a few ergs of inner energy available.

If you inhabit sensible, loose-fitting clothing and don't mind a little dust now and then, nothing you will need to do in a day to keep fit, get fitter, expand and simplify yourself, needs anything more.

It is probably useful at this point to consider a fundamental question: What are you going to do this for? Moral rectitude? I don't know any exercise vigorous enough. Flexibility? Strength? Stamina? Endorphins? Fun? Appearance? A long or happy life? The reason or combination of reasons for undertaking any program of fitness will determine what you do, how often and for how long.

A skeleton is loose. You can hold it by the skull and give it a shake and it'll rattle to beat hell. But people that tell you constantly to loosen up don't understand posture, at the very least, because if your bones rattled like that you'd be in PAIN. Something has to keep your bones from doing that — and from falling on the floor in a heap — and that something is MUSCLES. Be kind to them for they bear thee, literally, and they are your only defense against a myriad of ailments commonly thought to be the inevitable products of aging, including limited movement and fun, and endless pain.

The secret is POSTURE. And the secret to that secret is muscles in cooperative, collaborative TENSION. Of this they must remain capable to your last breath, not a difficult thing at all, but a thing nevertheless that requires some attention in this life of ease we have all slid into so EFFORTlessly.

And there, lurking innocently in that word up there, is the operative; it needs EFFORT. Only effort will keep you out of the ditch beside the road of life other happier souls are traveling.

Posture can be with you every waking moment, it quickly becomes a background thing and it begins to dawn on you that every moment is long and not worth overlooking. How are you sitting or standing right now, as you read this passage? Become aware of your spine, how you are holding your weight, where the center of gravity is, which foot you are favoring, what side is in tension, what in extension. See how things oppose each other toward a common aim, especially your back and stomach. Consider what it is that is Keeping You Where You Are.

It could be argued that being limber means being loose, but really if you study movement, organized, obedient movement, you find that it is the progressive looseness and tightness of the muscle groups, in proper sequence, that make a person well-coordinated and athletic. It is having a brain/body that knows the syntax of the movement and does not tense all the muscles at once, but makes them wait their turn and then instantly turns them on at just the proper moment to achieve the desired movement.

This can be accomplished with little muscles or big muscles, but they must be eager, ready muscles. They must be used to it, used to paying attention, and not flaccid, flabby things with poor blood supply, but well endowed, well fed and vigorous.

Muscles can be divided into two basic functions: FORCE, the amount of tension they can achieve at a given instant, and POWER, which is force over time, or ENDURANCE.

We all need some of each, but whether you need more of one type than the other is part of the question I first put to you: why are you doing this? If it's so you can hike all day, you need to favor endurance. You'll have less bulk to lift up all those hills, you'll go faster and easier with less expenditure of calories, oxygen and water, you'll breathe more easily and tire more slowly and be fitter at the end of a long day, provided you're traveling light.

But if you plan on traveling down dark alleys in the predawn madness, or lifting giant packs to the tops of mountains, maybe bulk is what you want. Even just as an intimidation display, for size, nothing beats the Lumps of Force.

How these differences manifest themselves in your day I will explain to you as we get down to your individual program.

Certain things are better done first in the day, and certain things are better done first in a given routine. Just as with language, there are semantics — the content of what you are doing — and syntax — the order and relationship of the parts to the whole. This is the language of motility, the beauty of a living, moving body.

We break a day's need down into manageable little chunks of no more than five or ten minutes. That way, when things get hectic later in the day, you will have the comfort of knowing that at least you did some of it. And kind of keep a little mental tally for tomorrow when, hopefully, you will do better; but it had better not always be tomorrow or soon you will realize, your body will tell you, that you have blown it.

N O T   E X E R C I S I N G

There is still a lot of day when you are not deliberately exercising, and a word about this larger time should perhaps come first, as being probably the more important. On the whole, the body was designed to walk well. It is poor at running for more than a flight to safety, though slow trotting can be fun, and it is poorer still at standing still. Don't do it much. If you have a job where you have to stand around all day, you probably already know this, and good luck at changing jobs.

Sitting has gotten a bum rap from nearly everybody, but to tell you the truth I can't see what's so wrong with it. It is leaning back that screws you up. Avoid chairs, whenever possible. In fact, furniture in general is designed to cripple us and make us uninteresting. Sit on the floor, or on a chair with your feet up or at least not leaning back (less in-your-face in public and about as good). And keep your spine straight; letting it round out in the lower back is a sign of weak muscles where you most desperately need them to be strong, and laziness, two forms of slow suicide. When your back sags, your will sags next.

Listen, this is an incredible, accidental once-in-a-lifetime opportunity— being alive— even when you think it's going shitty. If you can get up in the morning and ambulate, you are at least a minor hero to me. Congratulate yourself and get on with it. You have to cultivate the will to stay alive.

LIFE AND DEATH

Trying to define life is such a loaded concept, but let's start with something a little less controversial. Let me tell you what death is. Have you ever seen a dead person? A dead anything? If so, you know in your bones that DEATH IS PHYSICAL. Gravity wins.

Forget religion, forget airhead, chemically inspired breathless conversations with your enthusiastic kith and kin, LIFE, alas, IS also PHYSICAL. You like living? You want to keep on doing it for awhile? You need a body. You need to use it.

URGES

Habits, hunger and other irritations, are mainly just your body's reminder of what you did yesterday, and these impulses, strong as they can sometimes be, are not necessarily to be taken for intelligence. You have to be willing to push these feelings through the rational side of your brain, to understand where they come from, so you can expunge the ridiculous.

Also, when decisions are made, keep an eye on tomorrow. Whatever you do today, you're going to want to do tomorrow. Do you want to eat less tomorrow? Then relax, let the urge pass. It will, you know, and tomorrow you will reap the good karma. That's the way changes are made.

INGESTION

We could touch lightly here on the subject of ingestion: food, drink and drugs. During the day, as you wander the planet inquiringly, from time to time you notice other needs rearing their burdensome heads. And some of them, like air and water (hard to find in their natural state), sleep and food, and some place to deposit the by-products of all that combustion, are not going to go away unsatisfied.

I believe that, whatever you're contemplating ingesting, you have an obligation to try and understand the ramifications of what you are about to do.

D R U G S

INTERNALLY, drugs, including alcohol, are toxins, and the body tries as soon as they are ingested to get rid of them, feeling rightly or wrongly that A MISTAKE HAS BEEN MADE. In fact, some of the effects which might amuse our (somewhat) conscious minds may be attributed to all that adrenaline being stirred up in our body's defense against the dark invader.

EXTERNALLY, using drugs in some parts of the world means the powerful can cut off your head, or some other offending appendage you may subsequently miss, and throw the rest of you in jail forever.

The only legal highs that are probably quite safe these days are tea and coffee and, perhaps, beer. Too bad that leaves out marijuana, which might make you less obnoxious than beer, but travelers are realists, or turn

into them pretty quick, and you better know the
territory, as the Great Salesmen all said, if you want to
prosper in health.

Incidentally, if you want to use stimulants, ideally they
should be used against your natural circadian (daily)
rhythms, to even out your day. So coffee, for instance,
would best be taken in the midafternoon or after a
heavy meal, when you are liable to hit a natural low,
rather than in the morning, as westerners do, when life
is going to get you high, anyway. But life is hardly ever
perfect, nor does it need to be.

F O O D

When I was a kid, everything was Cowboys and ·
Indians. We played it day after day, when we weren't
inside watching Cowboy Movies on TV.

My brother always rooted for the Indians. I couldn't
understand that— the Cowboys had the neat hats, the
boots, and best of all, GUNS. COLT .44s, and HOL-
STERS. (Besides, they always won.)

But over the years, as I grew up, my allegiance slowly,
imperceptibly changed, until one day I realized it— I
was rooting for the cows. To me, killing animals is
patently unnecessary. I have lived vigorously and well
most of my lengthening life on vegetables, and prefer

canvas to leather as being lighter, cheaper, more comfortable and less problematic from the ethical standpoint. Lest you think I speak from a position of ignorance, let me add that I have tried hunting, fishing, keeping domestic animals for slaughter, and doing my own killing and butchering, and am satisfied it is cruel, as any child who happens by in the middle of a slaughter is likely to tell you (oh, you emperor in your fine duds).

Isn't this all part of fitness? Sort of?

MORNING

Okay, so you have survived another night, and hero that you are, you get up and head for the nearest depository. Then perhaps you indulge in the luxury of washing up, avoiding soap and other chemicals as just irritating baggage. Remember, we are light here, also thoughtful.

In general, I always try to think of a mechanical solution to a problem before bringing in the heavy guns, chemicals. When I was a kid, "Better Living through Chemistry" was gospel, thanks to the big chemical companies and their ad agencies. But I tell you, nothing has gotten a blacker eye in my time on the planet (except maybe "cheap" nuclear energy) than the chemical business, some of whose brainy ideas our great-great-grandchildren will still be cleaning up.

For hands, a little nail brush works as well as soap for most purposes— unless you've been cleaning your motorcycle or chimney, where gloves might have helped— and won't dry out your skin. And if you're worried about germs, you can forget it. The average healthy person has about two billion microbes on his/her skin, and every time you breathe a million more go in, too. Soap is not the reason you're healthy. Dishes don't need it, either. If you don't like the spots, dry them with a dishtowel (though I must make an exception for clothes, not being greasy things like us by nature). The planet will appreciate the chemical-reduced effluent emanating from your domicile.

If life lays a great, giant breakfast on you some morning, I hope you have the presence of mind to enjoy it thoroughly. But in general, don't do too much eating in the morning, especially anything sweet; it'll up your blood sugar and its expectations for the rest of the day and you'll never stop being hungry. Watch the heavy food too. That'll send the blood to your stomach, away from the brain you might need to plan your day.

Take it easy; look around. When you feel really awake, it is time for our first effort.

Morning is a lousy time to get strenuous, especially as a little experience begins to creep into your résumé. It isn't even the best time for serious stretching. So the first thing to do is a WARM-UP. Go outside, if possible and safe, go face the sun, the wind, the view, your shadow, or whatever amuses you, and prepare to accomplish something. This series is done standing, by the way. You can wear your finest baggy duds, but take off your jacket.

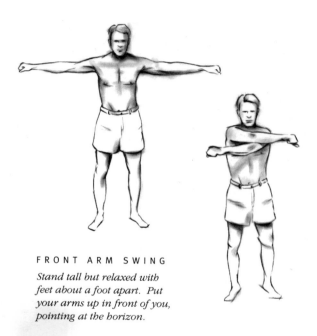

FRONT ARM SWING

Stand tall but relaxed with feet about a foot apart. Put your arms up in front of you, pointing at the horizon.

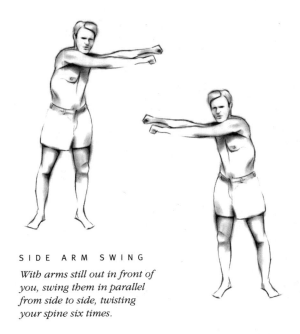

SIDE ARM SWING

With arms still out in front of you, swing them in parallel from side to side, twisting your spine six times.

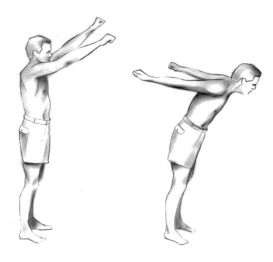

ARM ROTATION

Still with arms out in front of you, draw giant circles on each side. First, start down with your hands, coming up the back side and around the top, for six repetitions. Reverse direction of circles and do six more.

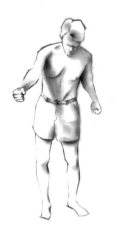
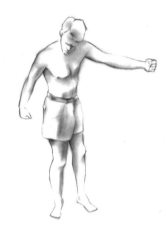

TWIST

Now we're going to twist; remember Chubby Checker and the old Dick Clark American Bandstand days? Never mind; imagine you're holding a towel behind you and you're going to dry your bum. Stand with your knees slightly bent and swing your hips opposite to your shoulders. Rotate with your left hip forward, at the same time swinging your right arm and shoulder forward, twisting your spine, your lower back; then, right hip forward and left arm and shoulder forward. Six repetitions.

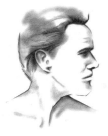

NECK STRETCH 1

Standing tall, turn your head left as far as it will comfortably go, and look out over your left shoulder. Hold for 6 seconds. Repeat to the right.

NECK STRETCH 2

Now, head forward and down, touch your chin(s) to your chest. Hold 6 seconds

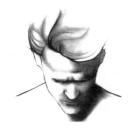

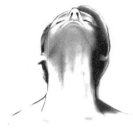

NECK STRETCH 3

Then head up and back, stretching your throat for 6 seconds (slowly; let's not induce a whiplash, here).

NECK STRETCH 4

Still looking forward, flop your head to the left, so that your left ear goes down toward your left shoulder, and hold for 6 seconds. Repeat to the right.

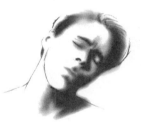

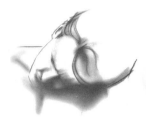

NECK STRETCH 5

Next, turn your face three quarters to the right while lowering your head down in front of the left shoulder; that's forward, down, with an opposite twist. Hold for 6 seconds. Repeat to the other side. You should feel the stretch all the way down to your shoulders.

SHOULDER STRETCH

This next one may be a bit hard at first, especially if you aren't endowed with long arms, but try putting one arm up behind your back, between your shoulder blades, then with your other hand, reach over the top and down behind your neck and try to touch your fingertips. If you can curl your fingers together, then you can really pull, and hold that for 6 seconds. Then go on to the other side.

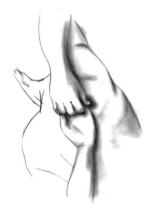

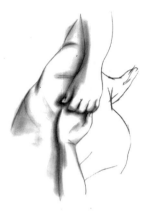

SHOULDER STRETCH

If you can't reach your fingers, go through the motions anyway; in fact, if you want to pull a little, grab a facecloth or towel and lower that down with your top hand, grab it with the bottom hand and, voila! you can pull, too, short arms or not, limber notwithstanding.

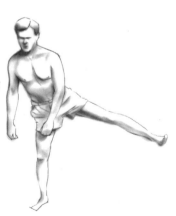

SIDE LEG SWING

Now, some lower body: Stand with feet close, still feeling tall, lift one foot off the ground and lift the leg straight out to the side, swinging from the hip. Do six repetitions. Repeat on the other side.

23

FRONT LEG SWING

Swing your leg up in front of you, as if kicking a ball, but take it as a stride, letting your arms swing, too; right leg up in front, left arm up in front, right arm back behind you. When you come down, swing right back behind you, as though kicking both front and back. Do six repetitions on both sides. Some people have trouble keeping their

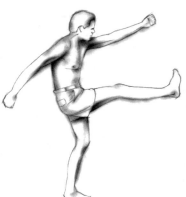

balance in these exercises, at first. Don't worry if you have to stop to catch yourself, just start up where you left off; you'll soon be doing it, no problem.

TOE STAND

Here's another one for balance, which is really just focus; these are actually mental exercises , but at the same time you're doing something good for your legs, ankles and feet. Bend knees slightly, stand on one foot, slowly lifting onto your toes, then back down, six times each side. As your heel contacts the ground, let your

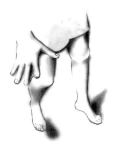

knee bend; if you let your leg spring, it's easier to keep your balance.

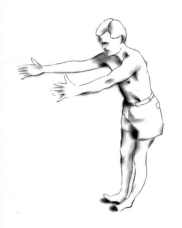

HEEL ROCK

Now we're going to rock both our feet together. Stand with your feet at least a few inches apart and rock up on your heels. As you do that, thrust your arms forward to help maintain your balance. Good for calves, ankles, feet, and shin muscles. Six repetitions.

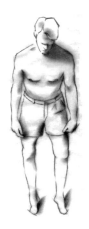 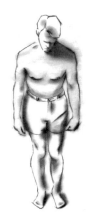

ANKLE ROCK

Now with feet about a foot apart, rock feet side-to-side; up onto the outside edges, then rock around until you're up on the inside edges of your feet. Do that six times, *but on the last of each, hold for an additional 6 seconds. Great for ankles, especially if you've ever injured them, and this is also good for the arches of your feet.*

26

BACK   STRETCH   1

*Here is the only occasion to
lock your knees (which you
shouldn't necessarily do; it
depends on how comfortable
it feels): We're going to swing
forward, but NOT from the
WAIST. Keep the small of your
back straight, make a little
concave arch in the small of
your back, a little lumbar
support— the real lumbar
support doesn't come from
chairs, couches and car
seats, never mind what the
ads tell you; the real lumbar
support comes from muscles,
okay? Those little muscles
have a lot they're asked to do,
so keep those straight, so your
back doesn't sag. You're
going to PIVOT from the
HIPS. Your knees are straight
(if comfortable) and you
swing forward from the hips,
just until your back is about*

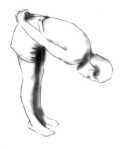

*parallel with the floor. You're
not trying to touch your toes,
you're not trying to get your
head way, way down by your
knees; all you're doing is
bending forward, your arms
behind your back, hands
clasped together. Now hold
that for 6 seconds with that
nice straight lower back.*

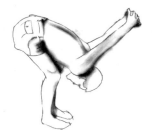

BACK STRETCH 2

Now bend your knees farther and lean forward more, while raising your arms up over your head as far as they will go, while still holding hands clasped. Let your chest drop down toward your knees and hold for 6 seconds.

BACK STRETCH 3

Now swing on down the rest of the way into a squatting position, heels on the floor, arms around knees. If you're used to this or pretty thin, you'll find your knees can go right up under your armpits. If you're heavier or have knee problems, don't try to squat down quite that far; nevertheless, you should attempt to keep your feet flat, heels down. Hold this pose as long

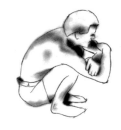

as you like, at least 6 seconds, but if it's really feeling good in the lower back or small of the back, linger, to a maximum of 30 seconds.

BACK BEND

As you start back up, again, go slowly at first; your knees have been asked to slide, they're not as simple a joint as people commonly think, and when you fold them up this much, they have to slide, and now you're ask-ing them to slide back, and some knees aren't too good at that, so START up SLOW-LY, lifting your thighs off your calves. Once you see your knees are working, just come all the way up and all the way over, leaning back-ward with your whole upper body, your hands clasped above your head, your elbows bent. Feel that in your stomach (but if you're feeling it in your back you've gone too far). Hold for 6 seconds, if you can.

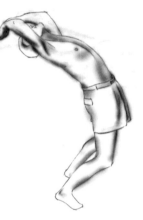

Some fitness professionals warn against bending your spine back at all. I think that view is a bit extreme, but you should listen to your body carefully, here.

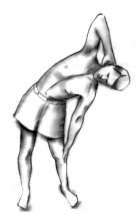

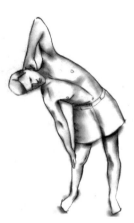

SIDE STRETCH

When you come back to the vertical, lean to one side, one arm behind your head, your elbow out, your other arm hanging down at your side. Bending toward the hanging arm, stretch your ribs, waist, hip, holding for 6 seconds; then repeat on the other side.

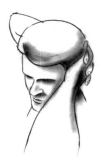

SPINE TWIST

That done, when you come back up, put both hands behind your head and turn your head so your left hand is cupping your left ear, giving your head about a three-quarter turn left. Now twist your whole body (except your feet) as far around as you can; get that spine twisting and hold it for 6 seconds, then swing around, cupping the right ear in the right hand, and twist around for 6 seconds on the other side.

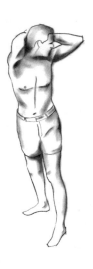

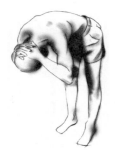

FORWARD BEND

With knees slightly bent, do six forward bends, remembering to bend from the HIP and not the waist. Keep your back straight and not farther down than parallel with the floor.

SQUAT

Still with feet in the same place, your hands hung down to your thighs, do six knee bends, feet flat to the floor. These aren't deep knee bends; don't go down too far, just till your thighs are parallel with the floor. As you go down, let your arms travel out in front of you toward the horizon. On the last one, hold it down for 6 seconds, if you can.

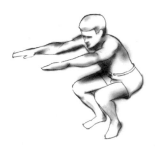

32

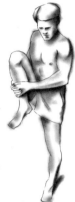

LEG TUCK FRONT

As you stand up, lift one foot and bring your knee up in front of you, wrapping your arms around your shin and clasping your hands together. Now pull up while you try to get tall, bring your knee in toward your chest, holding for 6 seconds. If this is hard on your knees, grab behind your knee, pulling your kneecap toward your chest but allowing your ankle and foot to stay out at whatever angle seems comfortable.

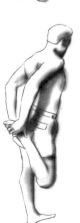

LEG TUCK BACK

Lower your leg, grab the instep of your foot and pull your leg up behind you. With your free hand, reach around and grab your toes and pull up, again holding for 6 seconds. (If you have knee problems, pass on this one.)

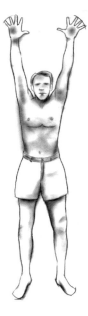

STRETCH

Raise your arms up as high as you can overhead and spread your fingers out as far as they will go. Get as tall as you can think, take a deep breath, and then exhale deeply for 6 seconds, feeling the stretch increase as you do, in your lower back, middle, then upper back.

That's all you need to do for now, but if you're eager and there's time— the whole world isn't waiting in the bus honking the horn promising unpleasant karma later— and you feel like more, roll on into the next small series (which only takes another minute or two): a general tensioning wake-up call to the major muscle groups, again done standing.

A point to remember on this one: NEVER HOLD YOUR BREATH. It can up your blood pressure impressively. Either exhale during tensions, possible with a six count, or breathe in and out, remembering during any exercise that the chest is like an accordion; when you expand it, it wants to suck in, when you contract it, it wants to release; so why fight it? (unless that's the point of the exercise).

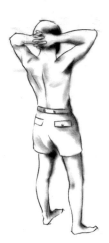

UPPER BODY 1

Bring your arms back down behind your head, fold together and pull forward with your arms, resisting with your neck, gradually increasing the pressure for 6 seconds; don't start out with a sudden leap.

UPPER BODY 2

Now, reach forward and put the heels of your hands on your forehead (above your glasses, if you're wearing any) and push back with your hands— and forward with your neck and head, to oppose— for a gradually increasing 6 seconds, until by the end of the count you should be pushing pretty damn hard.

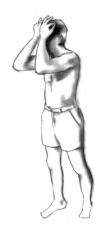

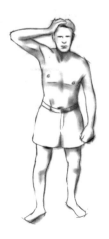

UPPER BODY 3

Now put the flat of one hand above your ear. You're going to push on the side of your head as hard as is comfortable and resist with your neck. Hold 6 seconds, then repeat on the other side.

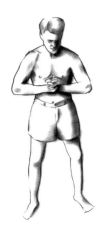

UPPER BODY 4

Now with your feet one or two feet apart, place your hands in front of your chest, heels together, and start pushing. Increase the pressure, as if you were trying to squish something in there, for 6 seconds.

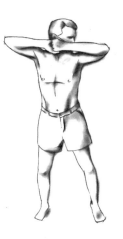

UPPER BODY 5

Turn your hands so the fingers cup each other and you can pull them apart; turn your head and hands so the back of your right hand faces your right cheek. Pull for 6 seconds, then rotate hands, turn your head the other way, so the left cheek faces the back of the left hand, and pull again for 6 seconds.

L O W E R   B O D Y   1

The next one involves a couple of things done simultaneously. Your feet are still apart, you're on good ground, in shoes that don't slide— because you're going to put some force into those feet now, and we don't want them to slide out from under you. Push your right foot outward to the right, your left foot outward to the left, tensioning the sides of your legs. At the same time, your hands are in front of you making fists, and you're going to squeeze your hands, to strengthen your fingers, grip, and lower arms. Hold that for 6 seconds.

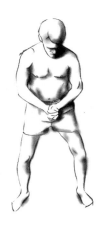

L O W E R   B O D Y   2

Now reclasp your hands with the other thumb on top and with your feet in the same position, try to pull your legs in toward one another, to get those inner thigh muscles, horseback riding muscles, for 6 seconds.

LOWER BODY 3

Now lift up on your toes a lit-
tle so your heels can swing,
and turn 90° pivoting to the
right until your feet line up
in series. Keeping your hands
together, put one hand on top
and the other underneath,
and push up with the bottom
hand while pushing down
with the top hand, so the
wrists oppose each other; at
the same time push the right
leg forward and the left leg
back. Hold for 6 seconds.

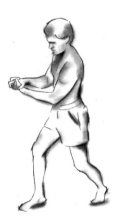

LOWER BODY 4

Now pivot all the way around
180° until your left leg is in
front and your right leg
behind, turn your hands over
so the other one is on top,
and again push for 6 sec-
onds.

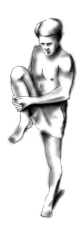

LEG TUCK FRONT

Okay, that's it; you've really tensioned every major muscle group in your body with that little one minute series. As a last move, before you walk away (because we're now done for the morning), grab your knee and pull it up to your chest, holding for 6 seconds on each side, just to stretch that lower back one more time. Now you're done until lunchtime, so go have fun.

A WORD ON REPETITIONS

This again bears on that first question I asked you: what are you doing this for? The MINIMUM useful number of repetitions for every figure is around SIX, unless you're not up to that yet, in which case even ONE is great, as it is on the unavoidable path to six. And six is also about right for you forceful types that yearn to bulge like bodybuilders. Turns out, thanks to the U.S. Navy who did the studies, six seconds at a time is all muscles can use for growth. After that you're just burning calories, noble perhaps, but beside the point in this context. You could save time by eating less. If you can do more than six repetitions of anything designed to tax a muscle, or hold any static tension for more than about six seconds, you will probably profit by making the exercise a bit harder.

If you strive for the middle road in general or aren't sure it's healthy to bulge so (it really isn't), TWELVE is more like it. This is a good compromise between force, that all-at-once strength, and endurance, that strength-over-time thing. There again, if twelve is too easy, it might be better to make the thing harder than to do more. But if you are determined that intellect and practical use will own the day, and there's time, THIRTY is about the extent you can go in tipping the scales toward endurance. Make the thing you are doing easy enough that thirty comes without killing you, and you will have struck a blow for freedom in our time. Women, who are usually partial to different bulges on their bodies, anyhow, seem to know this already.

Maybe you have, like me, some gross deficiency of form that is really bugging you (how impure!). Be of good cheer; it is not inconsistent to work different parts of your body for different goals, as long as your basic flexibility isn't compromised. Go ahead and beef up where you want; simply change the input of your program to change the result; just like a computer! Amazing, eh?

Be warned, though, that not all muscles show change at the same rate. Thighs can bulk dramatically in a month, (or shrink) while some other places take patience. You can either persist or at the least you will find out that it really didn't mean all that much to you after all— either an enlightening experience or a rationale for failure, you decide.

When it comes to STRETCHES, designed to lengthen the muscles and make them more flexible, THIRTY seconds is about the minimum for best effect. Don't bother with it first thing in the day, though, or in the program, as you can't stretch muscles very much until they have been heated up a little. That's why the warm-up, about six repetitions of easy stretches, comes first, followed by tensions that heat 'em up, followed by the really strenuous stuff, and finally, LAST by SERIOUS STRETCHING, when they can yield the most without risk of injury.

DARWIN IS WATCHING YOU

You may have noticed that as jocks get older they tend less and less to run in the early mornings. The reasons are really pretty Darwinian: the ones who always ran early have had proportionately more injuries than their lunch, afternoon or evening compatriots, and so less of them have survived to run another day. Why not take a lesson from these veterans now, when you are still young (or at least younger than you will ever be again), and give it up and get with the program, which is basically using your head to save your butt, and the Medical Plan.

THE DAY

Loose but not tired, stimulated but not stuffed, you are now ready for the day, at least part one of it. What should you do? As much as possible, WALK. Whenever time and space permit, your first choice should always be walking. This doesn't mean you have to walk the Atlantic (though I rowed it once quite happily), but you might consider walking to the dock or at least from the cab to the airline check-in counter carrying your own stuff. The idea is always to start with the assumption that you're going to walk and only abandon that after a genuine obstacle presents itself.

Bicycles are neat, fun and multiply your efficiency impressively, but when traveling they can be a little like traveling with pets: hard to get rid of when you don't want them, something to be guarded and worried over.

Shoes are simpler, with fewer moving parts, and less inclined (but not immune) to blowouts.

Be Eveready to take spontaneous advantage; much of life is adventitious and potentially Electrifying. Remember my casual reference to rowing the Atlantic? Well, the story is that I was on a first-class (sponsored) trip to Europe from New York on the Italian Line and after day one realized I was on a one-way pasta path to Gargantua's house, with nothing to do between the six meals of the day but read, pace the decks and do one-stroke laps in the miniature pool.

I love Italian food— fine, noble Italian food I could eat till I burst— and contemplating the next ten days with no sign of a storm to stop the endless feast filled me with a decadent dread. But in my relentless pursuit of places to poke my nose into and excuses to justify more eating, I discovered that next to the bridge the officers had an exercise room.

Great! They had stationary bicycles — good ones, and my first rowing machine. At the time I lived in a community, Toronto Islands, that banned cars but not bikes. I soon tired of beating the officers (good-humored as they were) at bike races and tried the rowing machine. It was love at first stroke!

Thereafter I spent a lot of time on the rower, gazing

out the big window at the sea rolling by. And I had the satisfaction of experiencing (sort of) the rowing of the Atlantic.

So keep your eyes open. There are more opportunities than time out there, at least as many as excuses.

MIDDAY

Sometime in the middle of the day you will probably stop for food, rest, to reconnoiter or to question your existence. This is a good time to really get physical. Rest for ten minutes or so, if you're tired. Have a drink of juice or something benign, but then press on. You can't be really worn out yet, the day is only half over, and what I am proposing, though strenuous, will only take a couple of minutes. It's time for your UPS. Keep in mind, as we discussed under REPETITIONS, what the thrust of your program is to be.

If you've been contemplating all morning and haven't done the morning warm-up, don't worry about it. In fact, it pays, in terms of general happiness, to remember YOU ARE NEVER BEHIND OR AHEAD OF WHERE YOU ARE. If it's noon, do the noon series. That's the beauty of doing a little often instead of a long routine a few times a week; when you miss a long routine, you really will feel you're getting behind.

The single most important UP is the SIT-UP. If you only have time for one UP, this is the one.

NEVER DO A STRAIGHT-LEG SIT-UP. It's hard on your lower back. If you can tuck your feet under something immovable and get your knees up high, you can really make this one hard. Anyway, for average conditioning get the count to TWELVE; for you forceful types, try to find a slope where your head is lower than your feet, maybe a lot lower, depending on how strong you already are. Or put your pack or briefcase or something on your stomach, and try to get the count down to SIX.

Endurance types can make it easier, if necessary, by leaving your arms at your sides instead of folding them under your head, or not raising the spine clear of the ground. But somehow, make THIRTY obtainable. As you all get used to this one, try on the last count to hold yourselves up, exhaling, for a static SIX count, as a little added test. You should fail or at least feel it.

As I said, the single most important UP is the SIT-UP. But if you are going to have time to do more than one, then start with the next most important UP, the PUSH-UP. Same numbers of repetitions apply.

Forceful types, you can make it harder, if necessary, by

putting something on your back (maybe a friend) or do them one-handed.

Endurance types might need to get the head-end up using a chair, stairs, a slope, log, or even the wall to make it easier, or pivot from your knees instead of your feet. Experiment, until the repetitions work out right for you, and again, you can add the little test at the end, holding halfway down for a SIX count, to make sure you've got the level of difficulty adjusted for your current potential.

By the way, varying the spread of your hands on this one will emphasize different muscle groups and can be surprisingly instructive and definitely make it harder.

The next one is sometimes hard to find a setup for, and isn't vital, anyway, but still feels great and uses different muscles, as you will find out by doing it soon after the push-ups and finding out you can. This is the CHIN-UP. Same count as before, but this time there is no easy way to make it easier; you are not likely going to do thirty of these, so try for whatever feels comfortable. But if you're after force and six is too easy, put your pack on or briefcase around your neck, or lift something with your feet, whatever it takes to make SIX the max you can handle. Again, try to hang on halfway up for an extra SIX count.

If you can only do one chin-up, or less, don't worry, you've got company. Like a lot of trucks that slow down going uphill, it's just your power-to-weight ratio. You can either shed some cargo or increase your horse-power, or both. And the way to do that is to keep on the program, keep pulling up even if all you can get off is your heels, secure in the knowledge that it will never be worse.

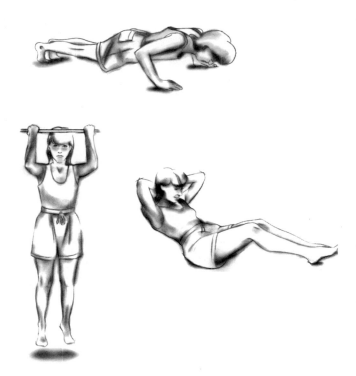

Okay, you're done, almost.
But the next time you see
something to walk under,
stop for a moment and do a
standing push-up: bend your
knees a little as you reach up
overhead and place both
hands on the lintel (upper
frame) or whatever is overhead. Then gradually increase
your pressure upward with
your whole body, especially
legs, arms and upper back.
Hold this for a six-count,
exhaling. (If you're short, try
to find something to walk
under just a few inches taller
than you are; but don't worry
if nothing presents itself, this
omission is also not life-
threatening.)

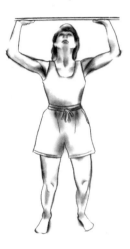

SWEAT

It may seem untoward to contemplate heavy effort in
street clothes, even business attire, but try it once. You'll
find out the whole thing takes less than two minutes
and you really can't sweat much in that amount of time,
no matter how hard you pull. Besides, moisture from
physical effort dries clean, no odor, assuming loose
clothing around your armpits. Believe it now, or after
you've tried it.

THE FEELING

I should mention what it ought to feel like, especially
for you bulking-up types. First of all, doing these exercises should never really cause extreme pain, especially
skeletal pain, such as in a joint or in your spine.
Especially watch out for pain in the small of your back.
Similarly, you should not feel burn in a tendon or ligament near a joint. The burn, if you feel one, and it
should be just a little, sweet one, must only come from
the center of the major muscle group being exercised.
Okay? Got it? Enthusiasm's great, but you can't do it all
in one day. It's a cumulative thing.

That's all. Go get some food, water or whatever, enjoy
the afternoon and we will meet up again one more time
around sunset. But remember, while you work your

way along life's trail, POSTURE! Relax but DON'T SIT BACK, and watch out for the sun, dehydration, cons, opportunities, nervous fatigue, confusion, communicable diseases, gravity, and political unrest, among other things.

TIME OUT

According to my body, there are at least six ways to sit. Some of them are good enough to sleep in if you're outside and afraid of getting run over, looking drunk, getting too much sun or rain, or getting jumped on by an unwelcome admirer.

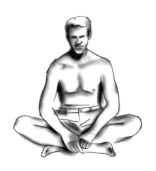

SIT 1

Try sitting cross-legged, your right leg in front of your left leg, and your right hand overlapping your left. Keep lower back straight and sit tall.

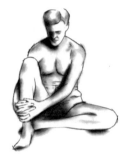

S I T 2

Now bring your right leg forward, clasping hands around shin. Watch that your lower back doesn't sag.

S I T 3

Bring both legs forward, arms around knees, top hand encircling wrist of lower arm. For sits 4, 5 and 6, try for the exact mirror image of these three, reversing positions of both your arms and legs.

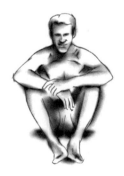

You can start with the basic position and move as you feel the urge through the series. By this time, you'll probably be tired of sitting anyway, but if not, the cycle repeats itself forever, like π, and you will never get stiff or sore, as long as you don't forget to move when you get antsy.

Feel free to invent more; there must be hundreds. Work with chairs, couches, cars or airline seats when necessary. Whatever's happening, stay off your elbows, and if you're driving with cruise control, keep a foot handy for the brake.

When you sit down from standing and again getting up, try doing it without your hands, even when you're just dropping into a chair. It's not really that hard, and it's good for balance, which is really just focus. But don't worry if you can't do it; it's omission is also not life-threatening.

We'd better digress:

THREAT ASSESSMENT

I divide life's situations into two basic categories, those which are life-threatening and those which aren't. If it's immediately life-threatening, mine or anyone else's, it's going to get my full adrenaline, my full attention, right now. But if it's not, then I'm not going to get too excited about it; it's more useful not to (and a lot more fun). When you run into something trivial, like just the imminent threat of incarceration, say, you can afford to take your time and watch developments a while, sit on your hands. It's good discipline.

You know, most of what humans do is unnecessary, anyway, a lot of it is harmful, and some of it is positively suicidal. (Could that be an oxymoron?) Feel the Amplitude of Time, as Whitman was fond of saying, its Amelioration.

YOUR ENGINE

You may be wondering about the old heart/lung machine, its care and feeding. Be heartened; it hardly needs anything. Like protein, strenuous exercise has been vastly overrated.

You need to puff and sweat. Yes, you do, but not for long. Not for anything that could be described as grueling or odious to even the most sedentary among us. To be precise (thanks this time to the Finnish government and in general the warmhearted and generous taxpayers of the world, who seem to have supported every fitness study ever done), you need SIX MINUTES a day.

So go walk briskly up a steep hill. Jump around. Chase a dog or your mate, skip imaginary rope or hop up a few flights of stairs — for all of which your cheap low-tech canvas shoes are ideal.

Swim, make love, or sweat profusely at a border checkpoint, having decided that they probably wouldn't search you for illicit substances — for all of which your low-tech canvas shoes are not ideal.

The idea is to take your pulse to about double the resting rate, and dilate those arteries. On the move it usually happens anyway. Even in the cities with all their conveniences, you'll often have to walk with your stuff. Hey, remembering it's good for you, you may even enjoy it.

EVENING

You've eaten, preferably early and preferably not too hugely; the middle of the day is a better time for that. I've found that evening is the safest time to indulge in a little sugar, if sweets excite you. Sometimes I just have the dessert I didn't really need at midday. It seems decadent not to get all the good vitamins and stuff every time you sit down, but I can testify that done occasionally it does not seem to be a burden to the system. Watch the whipped cream, if you're still into dairy. Sugar is a lot easier on you than fat, unless you're diabetic, though both are neurotic, I admit.

While we're on the subject of intake, let me tell you a well-kept secret about being fat. It uses up a lot more calories to sit around in a body of vigorous muscles than it does to sit around in a body of fat— I mean Sitting Around, Watching TV, Popping the Occasional Chip; Sitting Around Lazily Doing Nothing.

It doesn't seem fair, does it? Though they weigh the same and eat the same meals and largely do the same day, the athlete watches sports all weekend and doesn't get fatter, while the blob beside him does.

This is not just a macabre example of the Persistence of Memory. Turns out, it's not What You Weigh, it's What You're Weighing. Muscles are voracious, feeding all the time. Fat just sits there, waiting for the call.

It's not fair, but whoever said life was fair? That half hour a day you're putting in means more than you think. And that's your bonus. That's the real secret to getting thinner, permanently. Muscles. Effort. Physical Effort. You'll find out it's true: Life, alas, is Physical.

FLOORS

Now comes the longest workout of the day, still only about ten minutes, but not the most strenuous. For this you are likely to get dusty. These are the FLOORS, a lot of them stretches, after the usual warming, and once you are on to them, you are going to wonder how you ever got a real rest without them. These feel good; if the sunset is beautiful (pollution helps, here) and you can get outside, this is a fitting end to any day and I defy you not to smile when you're through.

Of course, if there is no outside or it's raining, there's always wherever you're going to sleep.

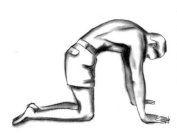

CAT 1

Get down on all fours, and raise up your back, arching it as high as you can, pushing down with your hands, and hold for 6 seconds.

CAT 2

Now make your back bend the other way, arching the small of your back and raising your head and buttocks as high as you can. Hold for 6 seconds. You should feel this in the small muscles on either side of your lower spine.

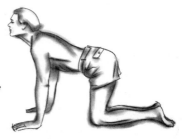

CAT 3

Turn your head and try to look behind you, stretching your waist and ribcage on one side. Hold for 6 seconds, then repeat on the other side.

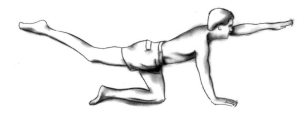

C A T 4

Now lift your left leg and right arm, extending them as far as possible toward the horizon, holding for 6 seconds. Repeat on the other side.

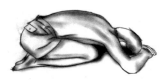

C A T 5

Slowly sink to the floor, letting your ankles, knees and hips fold up as far as possible. Hold for 6 seconds.

S T R E T C H

Roll over on your back, take a deep breath, stretch your arms overhead and spread out your fingers and toes. Try to get your toes as far away from your fingers as you can get them. Hold for 6 seconds.

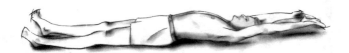

P E L V I C   T I L T

Lower your arms to your sides and with knees straight, rock the small of your back flat against the floor, tilting up your pubic bone. Hold for 6 seconds.

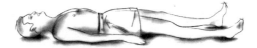

BUTTOCKS LIFT

*Now arching from your heels
and your upper back, raise
your buttocks clear of the
ground and hold for
6 seconds.*

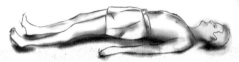

LEG LIFT 1

*Roll onto one hip, with your
arms out in front of you for
support. Lift both legs together
clear of the ground and
lower them. Repeat this from
six to thirty times, but on the
last repetition, hold for 6
seconds.*

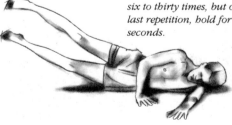

LEG LIFT 2

Take it easy on this one. On your back, put your arms under your lifted head, and with your knees bent, try to lift both feet off the ground and back down. Repeat this from six to thirty times, holding on the last repetition for 6 seconds. (CAUTION: You may have to bend your knees quite far, bringing your feet in close to your bum, to PROTECT the small of your BACK from stress.)

LEG LIFT 3

Roll onto the other hip and lift legs again six to thirty repetitions, holding for 6 seconds on the last.

LEG LIFT 4

Now on your stomach, try to lift your knees clear of the ground, with your legs slightly bent. Repeat six to thirty times, and hold for 6 seconds.

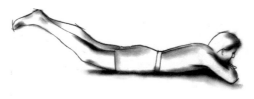

LEG LIFT 5

Now again on your back, with hands at your sides and knees slightly bent, raise your legs alternately overhead, fifteen per side.

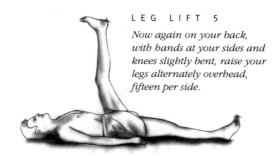

If you only have a couple of minutes for FLOORS, this is the series to do: the sitting cross-legged series.

CROSS-LEGGED 1

Sit cross-legged, your arms out in front of you, and start leaning forward, gradually easing your head down toward the floor, for 30 seconds.

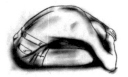

CROSS-LEGGED 2

Next, lean away from whichever leg is in front, cupping your hand under your leg and letting your head rest on your knee (if you can), your other knee held down by your other hand, for 30 seconds.

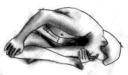

CROSS-LEGGED 3

Now switch legs over, so the other one is is front, and lean away to the other side, again holding down the opposite knee with your free hand, for 30 seconds.

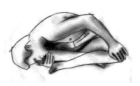

CROSS-LEGGED 4

Last, lean forward again, arms out in front of you, keeping legs folded as in the last exercise, and letting your body and head fold toward the floor for another 30 seconds.

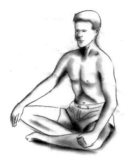

S T O M A C H   L I F T

Take a few deep breaths and then exhale once, deeply; then, with mouth and nose sealed against an inhalation, expand your chest and lengthen your spine, puffing out and sitting as tall as you can for 6 to 12 seconds. (Your stomach should really suck in on this one, if you're doing it right.)

L E G   S T R E T C H

Unfold one leg and lay it out straight, (knee locked, if possible) then grab your toes with the opposite hand and lean your head toward your toes (not your knee), stretching the back of your leg and buttock for 30 seconds. (I pull with my other hand on the side of the foot, to keep the tension even.) Repeat on other side.

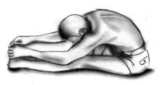

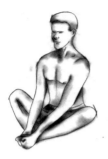

T E N D O N   S T R E T C H

Grab your toes and pull your feet toward your crotch, letting your knees float to the sides. Now rock the small of your back forward toward your heels and hold for 30 seconds.

S P I N E   T W I S T

Now cross your right foot over and place it on the floor outside your left knee. Put your right hand on the floor back behind you, resting it on just your fingertips, then weave your left arm, first, to the outside of your right knee, and then grabbing the top of your left knee. Now twist your spine around to the right and hold for 30 seconds. Repeat on other side. Try to keep both cheeks on ground.

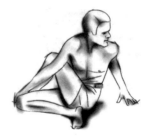

Let's assume that you have not been run over by a bus,
but have merely pulled a muscle or feel a twinge in
your knee one day. As soon as it happens, take the
strain off the part that hurts. Like any animal you should
instinctively want to favor the offended part, minimizing
pain. To minimize swelling, the standard wisdom is
RICE; Rest, Ice, Compression, Elevation. Try it if conve-
nient; if not, let pain inform you.

The next day, start with an assessment by doing the
morning stretch, carefully, and take it from there. You
may be surprised how much you can still do while
caring properly for the injured part.

This will help you to determine whether it's just a
muscle, which is quick to heel, or a tendon or ligament,
which is not so quick, or something skeletal, perhaps
even the onset of arthritis or bursitis or the like.

Or perhaps you know exactly what you did to cause
the injury and what is injured but still wonder how to
proceed, first, with assisting your recovery and second,
keeping the rest of you in shape while you wait.

As the days march on and you are trying to improve it,
it may be a little hard to define the line between just the
feeling of beneficial stretching and actual pain, which
really involves reinjury and may even amount to a new,

more severe injury than the original. All I can suggest is patience. If you baby it, it may never really give you back what it could, but if you overwork it, it may leave you with something permanently worse.

The stretching feeling should be extended in a very gradual way with no sudden movement or tension. Beyond that I can't tell you; you will have to learn for yourself. I have pulled a few bad ones in the process of learning on my body and believe me, if you do it, you'll know it right away; it hurts.

Of course, you can always seek medical advice from a doctor or physiotherapist if the injury seems unusual or confusing or severe.

ENJOYING

It depends a lot who you are. Some people's main problem will be boredom, a form of infidelity. Others will schedule themselves impossible tasks in the time available. But other than a quantum shift of focus, I can't prescribe for that.

I have been heartened to hear, finally, after thirty-five attentive years, a psychiatrist, someone in the Mental Profession, say unequivocally something I've always thought: It is a lot harder to be happy if one is not physically healthy. (Appropriately enough, this guy is seventy and has the body of a thirty year old.)

Besides minimizing the effects of time and keeping you happy and pain-free, there is another reason to take care of your body. Contrary to popular belief, the mind is not composed of the brain alone, but of a brain/body continuum, and the messages your mind receives from your body are a powerful component in your so-called rational thought process. Ignore the body, and the messages it offers up may just reflect your ignorance.

So a powerful case can be made for fitness legitimately assuming a high priority in your planning.

EQUIPMENT

We could talk clothing, footwear, first aid, the snail or turtle thing (your tent and sleeping bag) in the event you opt for self-sufficiency. The list of dangers while traveling might seem long but the spaces between them in reality are vast, and the great bulk of your time will be spent not in danger. So take heart, but take a few precautions, too.

For people awake in the daytime, black clothing is pretty dumb, though occasionally in vogue, except maybe seamen's sweaters worn where it's cold but crystal clear and not near dirt. Forget the stories you have heard about desert tribes in black robes, that only works if it's over forty degrees (centigrade), zero humidity, very windy and you don't mind looking pretty dusty. It's the wick effect; black heats up, you sweat into it (it's wrapped tightly next to your skin), the sweat is evaporated by the hot, dry wind, and this condensation of moisture causes a drop of temperature in the fabric. But when it dries out, look out.

However, if your wandering includes alleys in the pre-dawn madness (oh, you bulking types), sneaking around in black could be amusing, I suppose. Otherwise it's just a waste of weight.

Layers, as everyone knows by now, make sense, affording maximum flexibility for minimum stuff, and toward this end I find a thin long-sleeved collared shirt and a thick one better partners than a shirt and sweater; more comfortable, more pockets, you can wear either alone next to your skin, etc., (same for pants). But aside from general tips, like don't wear high heels, clothes are so personal you probably will work out your own ideas anyway. Baggy's the word, though, especially near glands, you'll be cooler in summer and warmer in winter, and your armpits (and other junctions) won't stink.

The One Rule: IF YOU CAN'T WORK OUT IN IT, LEAVE IT BEHIND.

Coats— ideally it should be coat— should cover all possibilities, from rain to wind to snow. I have what I call a one-coat I love (that great old vagabond cry for liberty, "One man, one coat!") based on an Australian horseman's coat but sewn of the very lightest weight Gore-Tex fabric and with a hood concealed inside the collar. This is long enough (it has reef points midway down to tie it up off your knees for hiking) to eliminate the need for rainpants and can be progressively closed in until it's as snug as a (movable) tent. But it flies behind in the lightest of breezes for brisk walking without sweat, and weighs so little it's like walking naked. It packs small, too— barely big enough for a pillow. Find something you can like as much as that, and you'll be a happy wanderer.

Shoes. I'm stuck with canvas, nylon cordura and the like, and light rubber boots, in my continuing effort to evade the enslavement of sentient beings, but this has not proved a particular hardship. They are available all over the world, cheap, are generally lighter and more breathable than animal skin footwear (if not as durable) and dry better after unplanned excursions into moistness. Buy them as you go; there's no blistery break-in period. And don't underestimate lightness. Clunky shoes, like black clothing, may occasionally be in vogue and give the impression of durability, but if they made airplanes that way we'd all be walking. Continually defying gravity is hard work.

Don't pack an expedition sleeping bag; you're never going to be where it's that cold, and anywhere else it's a real sweaty drag. I have a Gore-Tex mountaineering bag for Extreme People gathering dust, while my trusty old Canadian army bag with the flannel sheet insert and wooden toggle closures goes over its odometer for the third or fourth time. Tech is great.

PROTECTION

The obvious things to avoid are sun/heat stroke, dehydration, exposure (hypothermia), oxygen starvation (hypoxia) if you're in the high mountains, fatigue, including not getting enough sleep, and sex on the (quickly unzipped) fly, though some of you no doubt will indulge. Therefore, the condom deserves a place of honor in your medical kit (your wallet or purse is too accessible).

Also, speaking of protection, a HAT should be upper-most among your wardrobe as being better than the best sunscreen, more permanent, and less problematic (mechanical vs. chemical solution, remember). Ball caps are okay, but for serious sun they should have that romantic-looking, foreign legion-style cloth draping down over your neck and ears (a kerchief could serve) unless you have a lot of hair. Otherwise a brim is what is wanted. Lots to pick from. Keep it light, crushable, and ON when it's sunny, rainy, or cold in the vicinity of your head, which is to say, usually.

And try not to run out of money; being broke ups your worry quotient, which is a drag and definitely not health-inducing.

SAY GOODBYE

Altogether, you've invested about thirty minutes of your precious day, but this is the real housekeeping because this is the house you really live in, never mind what the neighbors think.

In fact, when I was young if somebody had come to me and said he would give me health and good cheer, freedom from pain (mostly), energy beyond my years, conditional insurance against premature demise and freedom from medical bills and pills and other quackery, all in return for no money and just a half hour a day, I would have traded prayer for sweat as being the better investment of time on the spot. Which is sort of what I did, come to think of it.

Take a day off now and then; I want you to miss me. There's more I could say, but we agreed to keep it small enough to take it with you.... So, BON VOYAGE!